Bits & P ve
Missed About e

ondition

by J King

MEDIA BOND elite publishers

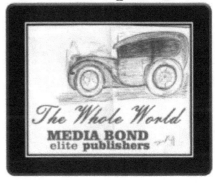

Table of Contents

To all those who encouraged it!

COLOUR MAP FOR REPEAT-BROWSING THE BOOK

Read what's written in **red** to review the book in 5 minutes.

Read what's written in **red** & **red** to review the book in 15 minutes.

Read the entire book to learn how to properly address your autoimmune condition.

INTRODUCTION

Autoimmune diseases are conditions that arise from an abnormal immune response against healthy body tissues. There are more than 80 variations of autoimmune maladies known. The immune system fails to recognize the cell's own antigens and attacks them. I felt this on myself since 2006, when I was diagnosed with Ankylosing Spondylitis (AS), another peculiar, draconic autoimmune case. After a titanic work and a set of extraordinary events, I have arrived to put it in reverse.

I wrote a book about it - *Ankylosing Spondylitis Killer, What worked for me,* which is currently helping patients of AS from all over the world. Ankylosing has a huge psychological element as the cause, and new scientific studies are finally investigating this. I then developed the section about this mental element for a deeper understanding in a second book - *The 7 Steps to Happiness, Ultimate Happiness,* because the results of what I had to mentally do to reverse AS filled me, on top of body health, with authentic happiness, and am sure it can do it for anyone.

Years of research, being a patient, talking to doctors, scientists, to other patients and being active on forums and autoimmune communities showed autoimmune diseases have more than the name in common. **While on the trajectory of the nerves anything can go wrong and the list of the +80 variations covers the widest area of effects and deformations possible, some of them even unimaginable to an ever-healthy person, <u>the reason the immune system turns against us seems to actually be the same</u>! Science is investigating this just now.**

The next rows include the relevant parts of the first two books, a condensed collection of analytics used in the findings, along with the set of instruments needed to address the root cause of the autoimmune flare, and not only the effects, thus fulfilling the role of personal recovery trainer. Don't be discouraged of hearing a lot about AS in the next pages, for in the end you will feel very much at home with what you've learned for your own autoimmune condition!

BACKGROUND

Suffering sure is a great teacher! As Dr. Abraham Twerski better puts it:

> *'The lobster's a soft mushy animal that lives inside of a rigid shell. That rigid shell does not expand. Well, how can the lobster grow? Well, as the lobster grows, that shell becomes very confining, and the lobster feels under pressure and uncomfortable. It goes under a rock formation to protect itself from predatory fish, casts off the shell, and produces a new one. Well, eventually, that shell becomes very uncomfortable as it grows. Back under the rocks. The lobster repeats these numerous times. The stimulus for the lobster to be able to grow is that it feels uncomfortable. Now, if lobsters had doctors, they would never grow because as soon as the lobster feels uncomfortable, goes to the doctor, gets a Valium, gets a Percocet, feels fine, never casts off his shell. I think that we have to realize that times of stress are also times that are signals for growth, and if we use adversity properly, we can grow through adversity.'*

While it is clear autoimmune diseases have effects on the patients' mental state due to pain, stress, and incapacity to deal with the condition, only recently, and here comes the novelty element, science (Donisan et al., 2015; Inderjeeth el al., 2016; Keith, 2018a; Keith, 2018b; Shmerling, 2018; Song et. al, 2018; Upham, 2018; Yurdakul et al., 2017) is looking into acknowledging the progression is opposite as well and, in fact, **mental disorders are producing auto-immune diseases too, and not only the vice versa!!!**

Abundant resources have been allocated over the last decades in researching the complex biological functioning of the brain, considering the physical factors were responsible for mental illnesses. That complexity is one reason that makes experts, such as Jerome Wakefield, PhD, DSW, a professor of psychiatry at New York University, believe too much emphasis is being placed on the biology of mental illness at this point in our understanding of the brain, disregarding the psychological implications. Decades of effort in understanding the biology of mental disorders have uncovered clues, but those clues haven't translated into improvements in diagnosis or treatment, he believes. *'We've thrown tens of billions of dollars into trying to identify biomarkers and biological substrates for mental disorders,'* Wakefield says. *'The fact is we've gotten very little out of all of that'* (Weir, 2012).

To be sure, sustains Wakefield, some psychological disorders are likely due to brain dysfunction; others, however, may stem from a chance combination of normal personality traits: *'In the unusual case where normal traits come together in a certain configuration, you may be maladapted to society. Call it a mental disorder if you want, but there's no smoking-gun malfunction in your brain'* and *'if we focus only at the brain level, we are likely to miss a lot of what's happening in mental disorders'* (Weir, 2012).

Thomas R. Insel, MD, director of the National Institute of Mental Health in the US, agrees – *'In most areas of medicine, we now have a whole toolkit to help us know what's going on, from the behavioural level to the molecular level. That has really led to enormous changes'* (Weir, 2012). Even though *'the diagnosis and treatment of mental illness is today where cardiology was 100 years ago'*, Insel adds, studies on hundreds of thousands of patients are already confirming the link between autoimmune conditions and mind due to the psychological factor being finally taken into consideration, and not only the biological one (Weir, 2012).

Yurdakul et al. (2017) explored the psychiatric disorders associated with my autoimmune condition, ankylosing spondylitis, and found **depression and anxiety is associated with disease activation, so not** only as effects of AS, but as triggering mechanisms (abstract of the study at the end of the book, in Appendix 1). Donisan et al. (2015; pp. 1345) further investigated the hypothesis that personality types could influence health-related quality of life (HRQol) using Jenkins Activity Survey, and the conclusion was: Type C and D personalities were found to be strongly correlated with decreased HRQol, and with higher disease activity levels, whereas type A was related to positive results in AS patients (summary of the study in Appendix 3).

A, B, C, and D types of personalities are concepts used in the field of medical psychology:

Type A personality generally refers to hard workers who are often preoccupied with schedules and the speed of their performance.

Type B personalities may be more creative, imaginative, and philosophical

Type C is the psychological disposition whereby an individual seems quiet and thoughtful but is in fact frustrated and angry. A person with a typical type C personality appears to lack emotions, and does not usually assert themselves. This type is associated with a greater chance of developing cancer

Type D is defined as the joint tendency towards negative affectivity (such worry, irritability, gloom) and social inhibition (e.g., reticence and a lack of self-assurance)

The medical system is living incipient stages of hunting authentic leads towards decoding autoimmune disorders! The answers expected from it didn't prove a viable healing option for me though, as they still move too slow. It's just reassuring, therefore the reason for mentioning them, that **studies backup my personal research, which also found AS is flared mentally.**

Here's how it all happened. The doctor told me AS is an autoimmune disease, a chronic, systemic disease, a form of rheumatoid arthritis, and a genetic disease, that it glues the spine, tenses the muscles and create inflammation on the trajectory of the nerves, and I will have to slow down its unquestionable future spreading with drugs, because the cure is not known, nor the cause. I understood in the early stages of the condition that it is not just a body issue and the solutions of the classical hospitals are not enough. Due to my former involvement in sports, I used self-control to interpret the body, I've put myself in a wide variety of biological and psychological tests, monitored and gathered results as a full-time activity. The findings and solutions came from an obsessive self-awareness of the body. **During the first years with AS I have tried to unnaturally keep a body posture, wrongly thinking that this is going to improve my situation. It didn't work, of course, it brought even more pain and stress, but it offered an even deeper understanding of the anatomy. I am now able to individually unstrain my muscles, even the peripheral ones, I can feel the tensions in the body and went as far as being able to link these strains with the moods and behaviours that are producing them. I was amazed too! When I was doing something mentally that I could observe releasing a tension in my body (due to my freakish ability, gained literally by mistake, of tracking nerve activity in my anatomy), I followed that path and felt unlocking the correspondent area in my back-then glued spine. The deeper I was going in understanding and controlling my mind, the better were the effects on the body. The more accurately I could perceive and discipline the oscillations of my thinking and their relation with the body, the more flexible and healthier I became. Everything tried was at first purely for body health, only long after to recollect what was actually happening to me, how my entire way of thinking and behaving changed, the impact of what I was doing on my personality and on the relation with others. I was so focused on my aim that I couldn't see the forest for the trees! Repairing my disease required to mentally heal myself first and escape of all insecurities and maladjustments to society in a very meticulous and organised way. Basically, I had to become really happy so I can be healthy, and only when I got healthy, I realised** how happy I am. From this angle, autoimmune diseases are an opportunity! Addressing them brings both mental and physical health.

It is an extremely systematic and diligent process. It is not a placebo effect or an attempt to induce an artificial mood. The result is crisp: the cause of having an autoimmune element is us, more exactly a combination of <u>7 specific harmful behaviours obsessively repeated together</u> (identified and explained in the *MENTAL CLEANSING* section of this chapter), assumed by most of us involuntarily, at an early age, from the toxic part of behaviours inherited from parents and in general from the environment we grew up in, from exaggerated self-blame and obsession with *I'm not good enough!*, from an unhealthy way of relating to inflamed thought patterns around us, leading to maladaptation to society, to inability of identifying and overcoming these patterns, or worse, and usually always valid, to deepening in them! <u>The +80 autoimmune diseases differentiate at core just by the distinct level of intensity in manifestations of one or more of the 7 behaviours!</u>

There are studies talking about injections that can activate some autoimmune conditions. The same injection is not activating the autoimmune condition in all people who are injected with it, but only to some, where there's already a body under the 7 behaviours and the injection unfortunately comes only as an immune system disturbant, a shock for the body, a mismatch, the last straw, allowing the condition to settle in easier and to suddenly be more obvious. Just as a metal is bending easier when being hit at a higher temperature than one hit at a normal temperature, the main reason the metal is bending is the hummer and not the heat.

I kept notes of each breakthrough and invested more and more time into it. That has been something pretty extreme for me when considering at the beginning I could be efficient mostly when alone and in silence. I have adjusted thinking patterns, tested myself between others, failed again and again until completely assumed the new healthy thinking and behavioural habits. That's when the rational arrives to be done from the heart and it becomes a natural thing to do. I read countless psychiatric, psychological and social studies, and been in contact with experts in the field, to make sense of what I was feeling, and kept track of my progression, to better understand what's happening to me.

There was a lot of struggles for this knowledge to be revealed and made sense of in these few pages. Tens of thousands of hours went into it and are at your click now. All autoimmune diseases sufferers who will cherish it and implement it wholeheartedly will be amazed. A whole new world will open up!

FINDINGS

MINDSET

I'm sure what I've just mentioned is something many might not be necessarily very happy to read, all the more the parents who are examining this for their children affected by an autoimmune malady and can observe a degree of responsibility for the condition they might've helped in being created (for example, when they tried, even with good intentions, to guide their child towards something specific, without fully taking in consideration who the child actually is, his natural inclinations, abilities, and limitations, and thus they might've created an artificial road for the kid, which could've raised confusion and rebellion in a sensitive mind). **The child might think he's not good enough and can become harsh with himself, too critical, turned against own person, just like the immune system turns against own person in autoimmune conditions!** These patterns can follow the child until much later in life and often the individual is not even aware of it, being so deepened in them and spending so much time in them that it may seem normal. But there's no place for despair - **Here lays the solution too! You did it to yourself in a way, you can reverse it too!**

For those totally dependent on the options now offered by hospitals and on other therapies that do not require the responsibility and involvement of the patient, a change of mindset will be needed for healing. **We are dealing with something far more complex than a purely biological disease!** The mental disorder is felt as a 'disconnection' between mind and heart, when people begin to live in their head, only partially really aware of what is happening to them and around them. The tumult creates destructive tension, harms and confuses the immune system, the inflamed thinking ends up being directly reflected in the anatomy and activates the auto-immune element. **The entire disease is activated by an obsessive overuse of the <u>certain</u> group of harmful** behaviours, both in thinking and in manifestation. There's a mental pattern linked to every disease in the body (besides viruses and other external factors of course), and when you know what it is you can begin to change the mental pattern so that you can change the disease. It is the body's way of telling us there is a faulty idea in the consciousness - Something that we're doing, something that we're believing, something that we're saying is not for our highest good! The body says - Please pay attention! When we know what these patterns are, a choice is again given to us: do we wish to do something about it or not.

Being such a personal thing to do, health seekers have to be ready to do it themselves, to take responsibility; that's when things start happening! A degree of complete honesty with oneself is required! And never stop educating yourself! Even just at a purely theoretical level, the effort of taking the situation in own hands, and at least understanding it and listening to others sharing the same experience, proves to be improving HRQol (health related quality of life) of patients, as with my AS, Inderjeeth et al. (2016, pp. 1134) found: AS Education Program in New York is effectively improving AS specific disease activity, pain and quality of life. Details of the study are shown at the end of the book, in Appendix 2.

Anyone with a bit of self-awareness already realises that bad moods are worsening their pain, while in good moods the pain is lighter. It's a matter of being present to understand it! Oh well, that's a continuous live event! Every single thought and attitude towards others, and life in general, is producing an effect in the physical body at any given moment. And when it manifests itself intensely and repetitively, the brain's getting overloaded and it disorientates the immune system. Now resolving it:

9

SOLUTIONS

I MENTAL CLEANSING

The way of thinking and addressing life must be changed and the unnatural nervous moods must disappear. The inflammation leading to the activation of the autoimmune component, and here comes the mind-blowing element, is created by the next harmful thinking patterns coming together at once, with an unfortunate triggering complementarity in their levels of intensity, for long periods of time, and on the background of an organism lacking basic detoxification: **1. Proudness, 2. Neediness, 3. Narcissism**, and, not less harmful, **4. Ungratefulness** (related to the upper back marrow), **5. Unforgiveness** (both on self and on others; hits the lower back), **6. Selfishness** (affects the whole spinal cord) **7. Dishonesty** (creates tensions in the middle of the spine, heart level). Call it a revelation or obsessive trying everything until discovering the game-changer, it is not a lucky guess. There is a deep rationale behind the findings, as I will soon explain, and addressing them incrementally, one leading to the other, is producing the healing from the root-cause, the one that ignites everything. The link between them (much easier to be understood once practicing them) dictates the relation of the individual who has them with other people and the effects of this relation. The link is shown in **Figure.1** bellow:

THE 7 STEPS TO HAPPINESS

RELATIONSHIP WITH OTHERS		FEATURE	EFFECT
1		PROUD	Getting lonely/ Disconnected
2		NEEDY	Flower that doesn't bloom for more than one day
3		NARCISSIST	Misfit
4		UNGRATEFUL	Dissatisfied
5		FORGIVING	Sunny
6		GENEROUS	Joyful
7		HONEST	Leaving in care/ No worries/ ULTIMATE HAPPINESS

The most difficult part is to communicate efficiently with an autoimmune disease patient, as he/she is already running an overworked and gloomy *software* (defective thinking patterns, chaotic brain activity, low attention and concentration). This whole period I came across hundreds, if not thousands of cases of stubbornness and angriness at new ideas, loss of hope, and pleasure of wrangle between AS patients (and in general between auto-immune conditions sufferers), outward accusation, despair, and a comfort in irresponsibility - *'others too are sick, the doctor says there's no cure, what's the point?!'...* an attitude of braking, of self-sabotage, just like our immune system becomes the enemy, precisely him, our doctor. It was very easy understandable for me, as I was part of the same team until a point; the big trouble is this kind of attitude not only it doesn't lead to recovery, most of the time it doesn't lead to even considering new solutions that work, and it brings depression and the feeling of giving up, which should never exist! That's also again understandable, as many of us have been so many times disappointed and given false hopes by hospitals or fake 'wonder-drug' sellers; it's somewhat normal to be skeptical. But let's not be complete eyes-shot in the face of our options. Regardless of how you address the disease, aim for full health and take yourself seriously! A serious condition asks for a serious resolution, it doesn't just go away with ibuprofen.

Those pain killers are tranquilising your behaviour, the mind is affected too. When full-health is the choice, the sick person can investigate how people who don't have pride, who are not needy, who don't have narcissism, unforgiveness, ungratefulness, selfishness, and dishonesty do. People can choose any solution they want, and believe it's working, to test it and reverse the behaviours. They will realise that **all solutions are going in the same direction, specifically into practicing the exact opposite behaviours of the harmful ones:**

The answer to vice (prison)

is virtue (freedom)

1. <u>Instead of pride, they will have to open their ears more to others'</u> <u>knowledge and opinion, and to associate their own good deeds and</u> <u>talents to their native gifts, chances, and environment as well, which</u> <u>are not necessarily their merit.</u>

Who is here? Arrogant persons only hear themselves, consider they are above others, despise others, are insensitive and cold. They have a rubber attitude. As rubber isolates electricity, they isolate themselves from learning. They always find justifications for their wrongs, and this way they always remain in the blind. They are an unpleasant company and will soon be avoided. **They will remain lonely. And this is usually the wake-up point, the trigger that makes them trying to surpass Step 1. When they remain too lonely, the only way to get friends is to start becoming a friend, so they will have to do something about themselves. Proud persons, in this sense, present themselves as much better than they are. This is a soil for countless mental disorders, when disconnected so far from reality. They deprive themselves of the abundant knowledge and guidance that surrounds us, completely missing the whole game.**

How to overcome it? No one is better, we are just different. We each have different gifts and different limitations. Imagine the multitude of knowledge and opportunities from all these gifts combined. Proud people can understand none of that. How can they be sure that someone they disregard wouldn't blossom more than them if that person would have their gifts, chances, or misfortunes?! To conquer this Step, people here must start allowing a degree of self-emptying themselves, and they will have to listen more and learn more, to allow life to enter in their bubble environment they wrongly created for themselves.

What is the gain from overcoming it? It will make them finally understand we are social beings. Between people is good, is where wisdom, educative challenges, opportunities, and rewards are. They will soon realise there's much more to life than they knew and they will instantly feel livelier, like just woken up from the dead.

♣

2. <u>Instead of being just needy for others' attention, they might consider seeing their own worth (good parts and also limitations), without seeking others' approval</u>

Who is here? The situation is a bit ameliorated compared to Step 1, with people being more connected to society, as here there is the actual need for others. Only this need is for harmful use, to sustain an image without background. The persons working Step 2 need the others to constantly be approved by them, otherwise they feel empty. The persons here depend on others' attention and cannot breathe by themselves. As they leave the overwhelming solitude of Step 1, they fall in the opposite extreme, and they do not understand that silence and solitude can be good at times. It is very normal to be needed in society, to be respected for who we are and what we do, the illusion in question here appears when people are detached from who they really are. **They are insecure while presenting themselves tough, they are often playing an act, and their reality is the other's approval, which helps them feel good, but not for more than one day at a time, often struggling with disappointment and depression. This is also a productive soil for mental disbalances.** However, the persons at Step 2 made progress from Step 1. They are a little bit more down to earth here.

How to overcome it? The healthy way is, again, to practice the opposite behaviour of the one that's been identified not doing good to them: to spot own limitations and abilities, to begin putting the abilities to work, to get the courage to start changing what can be changed, to accept with serenity what cannot be changed, and to thrive for the clarity to make the difference between the two.

What is the gain from overcoming it? This is the beginning of understanding the existence of own identity, of integrity, and will offer a preview on the power and peace of having it well-defined can bring. Those who know themselves are winning everyone around them. Moments between people will offer insights about their own identity. They will observe the way they manage themselves while relating to different types of people, and this will give them insights about their own identity, about its uniqueness, and about the need of this identity for the environment they live in.

♣

3. The opposite of narcissism is being empathic

Who is here? The situation ameliorates further, people around are seen as more and more important, but persons affected by it are still in a very dark place. Exaggerated self-love, in the sense of narcissism here, is in itself a recognised personality disorder, characterized by a distorted sense of self-importance, need for admiration, and lack of empathy. **They promote an illusion and they demand others to pretend it is real.** Narcissists are frequently demeaning, they intimidate, bully, and exploit others without guilt or shame. They are misfits. They live in a fantasy world that supports their delusions of grandeur. **Compared to Steps 1 and 2, the people here have a higher sense of appreciation, people around them start to mean even more and to grow in their eyes, but they do the same mistake of using the breakthrough wrong. They need the others not only to receive attention, as at Step 2, they now demand to be loved.**

How to overcome it? To conquer Step 3, people here must practice empathy. Empathy is the capacity to understand or feel what another person is experiencing from within their frame of reference, that is, the capacity to place oneself in another's position.

What is the gain from overcoming it? This is good progress from the previous step: they now have a concept of love, even if it is a crooked one. We slowly move away from acute mental disorders and this will be felt by those around them, which will make people at this stage fit in better.

4. The opposite of ungratefulness is gratitude for whatever life is throwing at them; there's sure a lesson to be learned from any situation

Who is here? The appreciation for others grows even more at Step 4. The former narcissists understand here their illusion is not sustainable and start to sympathize with other people more. It's almost like others are as valuable as them now, but still not quite so. They still feel they are entitled to more than others. Even though there's finally some sort of more balanced social life, the ungratefulness gives them in the background the sour taste of dissatisfaction. Ungrateful persons have hearts that cannot be compassionate.

How to overcome it? Of course, with gratitude; gratitude for whatever life throws at them. That's the positioning from where people start accepting the game of life and take responsibility for really doing something to manage it well, as they see there's much to be gained from it.

What is the gain from overcoming it? This brings significant rewards as they now start loving to play the game of life. They are less and less dissatisfied. Gratitude opens many gates. There is much less struggle and they move towards the sunny side. The persons who conquer Step 4 become grateful. The grateful persons are good members of society. They have a healthy mind, a good heart, and a soul devoid of cunning. It's easy for them to become friends and make friends. They wake up satisfied and embrace life in all its complexity and unpredictability.

♣

5. <u>The opposite of unforgiveness is to simply forgive, both the</u> <u>others and oneself.</u> <u>This way people move forward with ease</u>

Who is here? Unforgiving people feel as they are carrying an extra weight on their shoulders. They are always looking for a culprit to their suffering. They have the need to be right and they put that before peace, when in fact **peace is greater than being right.** They don't allow themselves to be free from the tensions unforgiveness comes with. It feels like there's a string between them and the person they don't forgive, like their free movement is restrained. This doesn't let them manage their life with ease and move further. **They drag with them consciousness grunge and grime they cannot explain, as they don't understand yet the immense rewards of forgiveness.**

How to overcome it? The only way to pass this is to forgive! To forgive is to love, to love someone despite his guilt, no matter what the guilt is. It's not just superficially throwing a sorry in there. It's the act of completely cutting the harmful psychological chain with the person that has done wrong to them. And in fact, it means to be responsible for oneself. People need to do this for themselves, for their own good. Forgiveness is a choice. After forgiveness comes reconciliation, then healing. No one is better than the other. Everybody does the best they can with the skills they have. Familiarity is not good! We each only represent ourselves. When people finally understand we're all a bit coo-coo in the head, life becomes much easier. We all do

mistakes. And we can all be forgiven; we just have to ask for it.

What is the gain from overcoming it? Arriving here is huge progress. A constant good disposition will wrap the heart. Not being tied with any chain of unforgiveness and criticism lets people here flow freely through life, accepting all events with a sunny spirit and a learning mood. They now move from being just satisfied with life to being sunny. People here start to gather a lot of joy and they don't always know what to do with it, so, feeling free from the others, they invest more time in themselves and in their passions.

♣

6. The opposite of selfishness is altruism, discovering that putting others' welfare before theirs brings more benefits

Who is here? The selfishness in question here refers more to the unsharing of the sunny state achieved when passing Step 5. People at this stage appreciate others and they appreciate life, they make time for themselves and their projects, and still remain with some time and joy they don't know what to do with. They are joyful but they don't feel complete. However, they feel they are on the verge of something big.

How to overcome it? When people here burst of joy and they have already so many skills climbing the first 5 Steps, the next thing to do is to share that joy with those around them, to be generous in any way they can. Others might benefit from their word, or from their listening, or even only from their presence.

What is the gain from overcoming it? The reward will not take long to appear, as in the saying *what goes around comes around*. And this is even more accentuated when it's about a superior connectivity between people, such being forgiving is. This will make people feel meaningful in society, and that will bring them joy. They will wake up wanting to *play* life together, knowing that what they do every day in relation to others have an impact on their own lives. They will realise it's more pleasant to give than to receive.

♣

7. The opposite of dishonesty is clearly to never lie, neither to others nor to self

Who is here? Here is the last threshold that some people struggle to understand it even exists. People here embrace life. They spend time in helping others and they understand the naturalness of it. They see the rewards of such deeds and how life embraces them back and takes care of them when they do good, or some losses appear when they do bad, but they don't try to understand more about how is that possible. They lie to themselves, most of the time without wanting it or questioning themselves, that this area of research is unapproachable. But who does that? What are these exterior organised forces that take care of them when they do good or help them sabotage themselves when they do bad? They start observing 'coincidences', which they cannot explain, nor try to make sense of. This happens more often to people here and, although they acknowledge it, they don't go further in trying to learn more about it and they prefer to remain just worldly, terrestrial, to what they can see only. In the expression *What goes around comes around*, the *goes* part is up to us; what many disregard to think about is the *comes* part. They take it for granted instead of studying it. Dishonesty refers here to the refusal of examining the liveliness and wisdom of the exterior support they observe they get when they do good, as well as the maleficent of the other forces from which they notice it's coming even more harm when they do bad. They can see at this point how clever and well organised this exterior support is, but they act like it's something automatic and inexplicable. They lie to themselves that what they know is a complete view. The persons here gathered already plenty of understanding of life, but are struggling with this exterior support, as it is mostly invisible and seems hard to make sense of, even though they completely acknowledge its work. So, most often from atony and commodity, they close the eye to trying to find an explanation for it or to learn more about these forces. Some are calling them universe, some God and evil, some nature, whose work for the persons here is obvious but not yet explained.

How to overcome it? Instead of closing the eye and lie to themselves about this particular subject, persons here will have to think about the cleverness of all the factors in their life that brought them where they are now and were away from their control. They will realise there are a lot of well organised factors from the exterior, correlated in time, such as 'coincidences', a message from a book that came in the right moment and resolved a situation, the appearance of a person in their life that made them learn a lesson due, a disease that hit them and after overcoming it left them with a set of strengths that helped in more areas of their life or, in the opposite direction, some voices in their heads pushing them to do something that they then regret and can't understand how they were able to act like that in the first place. The external influences feed what we put our will into: the good ones feed the good, the bad ones feed the bad. These influences have an intelligence to them and are not just random. People here already have a lot of social experience. Now it's simply the time to stop depriving themselves from answers to existing questions, to dare looking for explanations to what they've already observed, until they find them. How did that happen? Who's behind them? Those who seek find; the forces are constantly in the phone receiver, waiting just for our choice. Seriousness in the inquiry is vital, as also in the testing of the findings, so that can be made the difference between false and real, evil forces being always busy presenting broken forms of truth as 'authentic', and some people might encounter those ones first in their research, before the real thing. Only one can never disappoint though, being absolutely perfect, and that's when the explorers succeeded.

What is the gain from overcoming it? This is the last piece of the puzzle. The picture of the *life game* is complete. Absolutely everything is taken into consideration now. People who climbed to arrive here understood the constant battle and its gains, they assessed the needs and they constantly reached for solutions. The understood the effort and its rewards. They understood that when the effort is put to work for the good, there is a superior intelligence of life which is rewarding, clever, and alive, that encourages this path. And when the effort is used for the bad, there are some forces encouraging that path, 'helping' towards self-sabotage. This starts from people's thoughts, the impulses/'voices'/thoughts in the head that all speak with our own voice, but are not actually all ours. Ours is the freedom to choose between them. People arrived here can discern between the 'voices'/thoughts (*good*, *bad* and *own*), and choose to work together with the good ones, as they become aware of their assistance, guidance, encouragement, protection, and relief. They get a sense of spirituality, of understanding how the unseen works. People here master their game. Having discernment, they observe the most suitable path for them, being now illuminated by the good force. Everyone's endowed with the ability to discern between good and bad. Sometimes this discernment is distorted by our passions or by mental illnesses. The distinction between good and bad can be further distorted by externals. Our perception is limited to what we see, but we do not know what is in a person's soul. The gift of discernment is to acquire the eyes of those good forces, who look at the inner man, at the heart. Further, we do not see where a person's actions or decisions may lead, but those good forces foresee all things. The gift of discernment is mainly the acquisition of the 'eyes' of those good forces, which look at the inner man, at the heart, knowing better than us and wanting even more than us what is good for us, but choosing to create this good only if we want it too. Discernment in full has 3 stages: know the self, acquire the 'eyes' of the good forces, and know those force's will. Those arrived here gain an understanding of the full spectrum: individual, society, and higher influences. This makes people aware, mature, which brings a sense of accomplishment and completeness. They can now face with calm any material or nonmaterial challenge, knowing life is more than the seen part, and in fact everything adds up in the personal accomplishment depending on the quality of the relation with those forces. Everything is made for a supreme good of ours, even if not completely understood by us. <u>Nothing happens without the will of the good forces or without their permission. They rule! WE ARE LIVING IN A UNIVERSE UNDER A GOOD REIGN</u>! The measure of goodness takes place in each person's heart; most definitely not enough hearts are gathering this goodness, from here the state of our macro-society today. These forces are noble and they respect our will, even when we choose the bad. <u>As powerful as it is dangerous, we have the freedom to choose between good and bad forces</u>. Whenever we have a rebuke of conscience and we experience *fear, turmoil, anxiety, despair* or we are possessed by *hatred* and *envy*, it's because we are <u>definitely</u> allowing a dark spirit in our life through our bad choices towards its bait. <u>We are responsible for that!</u> And <u>we can be sure we're</u> with the good forces when there's *love, joy, peace, kindness, patience* or *good deeds*. We are always stepping up or down on the ladder, as we are always vibrating more with one of the two sides, attracting it. <u>We are never still on the ladder</u>. The persons climbing *the 7 Steps* are aware at this point of their advantages and limitations, they feel at full potential, understanding the good is coming from caring for others, and that everyone deserves to be treated with the same love, as this is also what the good external forces are supporting. Zooming out, to see the full picture, the complete reality, we are coming with the will and the work, and when we choose to partner with the good forces, they are coming with the protection and the wisdom! It's a dynamic process, live, a partnership! The more we allow the good forces to be part of our lives, the more we are contemplating the marvellous development of events and the less we worry. <u>When we don't think much about ourselves everything goes well! Something incomprehensible for those at inferior steps becomes a lifestyle for those on top of Step</u>

7. That's what keeps a clean, happy, worry-free mind, and no mental nuisances will touch that. That's the true nature of the mind! That's where Ultimate Happiness is at home!

♣

You can get bored or tired of self-developing yourself, but for someone else's smile there are always easy-to-be-found resources, and it's more rewarding to do things for others. There's a higher knowledge here; it doesn't mean that you have to neglect yourself, the opposite in fact: the more you want to be there for others, the more peaceful you first have to be yourself and the more vigilant you have to be at your own game first, so you'll make sure you'll offer the help needed and not just something you think it would help and in reality, it wouldn't. **An understanding of others comes from an understanding of oneself. And helping others in this way leads to be helped by these exterior forces in amazing, inconceivable fashion. If you really want to help someone you have to only see the good in them, to address that good! From here the dimension of the bubbles and their progress in Figure 1. To be happy is to make others happy first. This opening of the heart is done by gratitude for the work of these great external forces, through deep sorrow towards our bad moves or to put ourselves in the situation of those who are in trouble and suffer with them.**

For this mental recovery process, some people have results from introspection, some from talking to friends about it, some from reading a lot about it, some from going to psychologists, some from drowning themselves in the physical work, dancing or sports that they like, which calms down the mind, then acting sharper on the steps. Constant education is a must, to train and feed the brain and the soul as you train and feed the body. There's now easy access to a lot of useful information. **The best way I came across is to do it as Christians Orthodox do. They have the Confession (they tell God in front of the priest the bad thoughts/paths/inflamed ways of thinking), which cuts loose** the past chains of harmful behaviours, hence the bad habits; then they have the Communion (actual unification with God, with those good external forces), which helps in establishing the new healthy behaviours, together with the ongoing will of the person to change for good, both thinking and doing. The stillness they then practice in front of the icon and the short Jesus prayer are gold for both the mind and the heart, thus for the body, with immediate effect on the nervous system. They have the good forces' direct solutions on their side. The huge impact of this *prayer of the heart* (done under guidance) on the nervous system is widely recognised in Russia and Greece, where doctors are recommending it to their patients. An introduction to this subject can be found in the book of Kallistos Ware - The Orthodox Way.

The focus is to train, in any way found effective, the exact opposite behaviour of the one that produces harm. That's the deepest, most sustainable, and fastest way of addressing a faulty mind, the root cause of all unhappiness!

Arsenie Boca explains in his book - *The Path to the Kingdom*: '*The diseases appear in the energetic field of people years before they manifest in the physical plan. The disease comes from the soul and not from the body. Suffering is started upstairs, in the mind, from the conception about the world, from the mental imbalance in which we wander. - Hey, for those narrow-minded there's no cure!*' (More details in Appendix 6).

And once more, an extract from the book *Mother Gavrilia: The Ascetic of Love* (2008, pp.426): '*Behind any disease is a pain of the soul. Nothing bad happens to the body when the mind and spirit are healthy. It all starts with worries. Nowadays all doctors know this... The disease begins in the mind, with a negative thought, through a constant unrest*'.

Figure 2. below is more of a general representation of consciousness and can be used as an individual check scale - the more expanded the consciousness, the more authentic the person feels and less mental disorder is experiencing.

26

Looking at the map in Figure 2, and considering the time already spent with the disease in HYPERACTIVITY and INACTION zones, autoimmune diseases cure in the POWER area, with a constant flow from REASON upwards. It can be useful to have a general self-check with Figure 2, and then to spend time everyday working around Figure 1.

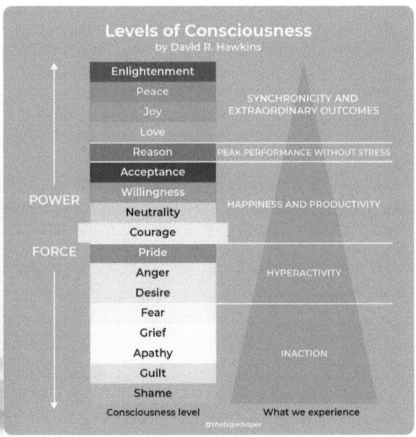

The next solution turns out to be an ally of the mental cleansing process. It's a powerful state-of-the-art technology that biologically boosts the entire body and physically sharpens the mind. Even though it is not directly addressing the psychological element, it can go as far as cleaning the neurons from toxins, thus having a considerable impact on the behavioural experience.

II BIOELECTROMAGNETIC THERAPY

It is a non-invasive computerized therapy. Basically, any harmful virus, bacteria, and parasite known to man has a resonant frequency. A good clinic will have a database with all these frequencies. The doctor will move an antenna around you and will immediately be shown in the system all the stuff you shouldn't have in your body. Those are creating blockages and are not letting your immune system to be able to do its job of repairing the body.

In the treatment part, to the patient connected to the computer are sent specific anti-frequencies to cancel the existing biologically harmful elements. Depending on the advance of the condition, a different number of sessions could be necessary, at a distance of 4-8 weeks, sometimes more. **This technology is spot on as it is able to custom the diet for each body,** and not just a generic menu for one disease.

After the visit, the temporary, but very strict diet will be given (I had 41 foods banned after my first visit). Specific supplements (usually plant-based) are prescribed to also attack those blockages and to encourage the weakened components. Between many others, I have been found with dilated neurons, with holes in them where toxins were gathering, and hyperactivity in the parts of the brains related to inflammatory behaviours, plus migration of calcium from bones to organs.

All three together (diet, supplements, and clinic treatment) are releasing the immune system, the balance will start to be regained in the body. In my case the lungs began to breathe better, the hear

to operate smoother, and, most important, it makes the mind more supple, thus enabling it to choose more accurately and rationally the thoughts, and not just randomly from the amalgam of mental scripts an inflamed thinking comes with. There are clinics with complete frequency databases in the US, Australia, Romania, Portugal, etc. Effects can be felt immediately after starting treatment.

It has now been a century since the technology was firstly introduced with good results by Georges Lakhovsky in France (Rogers, 1996). This kind of therapy is not making money for the pharmaceutical industry, which is why it is not in the mainstream. However, the results of the magic resonant frequency, as it is called, are obvious (more on Resonant Frequency in Appendix 7). It feels like a deep internal wash, at the cellular level.

Those for whom a visit to such a clinic is inaccessible will have to take care of their diet as elegantly as possible, carefully identifying and eliminating foods and drinks with inflammatory effects, which visibly make them more anxious, those that worsen the disease and lead to more stiffness, bloating, cause redness, itchy skin, ignite psoriasis, or whatever other way your autoimmune condition is expressing itself! This will make a major difference in the way the mind works too!

I was given powdered milk when I was a toddler, then I ate messy, with excess gluten, sugars, etc. Those foods did not lead to AS, but they weakened the resistance force of the body and mind, allowing the disease to settle in easier.

29

III FASTING

This method is an upgrade of a detox diet and after trying it the rehabilitation took a way faster pace. I only drank water, without having any food, for 13 days, and detoxified with enema. The memory of the drastic change and the confidence in recovery I got at that stage pushed me ever since.

I have convinced myself to try fasting only with water by reading *Fasting*, a book by Thierry de Lestrade. **After 48 hours without food, body functions are subservient changing**, protein is saved in order to keep the muscle of the heart pumping and the body firstly burns the unwanted and non-vital deposits. Not only I experienced something that I would call a rejuvenation, it mentally felt like I've just installed a new, fresh operating system. I've lost 10 kilos in 13 days. It initially started as a 3 days experiment but I continued until day 13 because it was so easy and effective. I am repeating it since, most often with one 5-days-session every two months, and 3 days of each week I'm eating vegan. Recently I've done it for 21 days, and the effect is proportional.

Physical hunger passes after the first 2 days and it remains only a mental appetite, activated by seeing other people eating or watching food adverts on TV. The body announces when the physical hunger returns, just like the indicator on a car when it's out of petrol but can still go for another 40 miles before being empty. That can happen after 2, 3 or even 6 weeks to some people, and it would be a *full service*, a complete fast.

The change in the body is very complex and the flexibility gained in such a short time was more than surprising. My mind got so peaceful!

For those older amongst us, those on heavy medication, and those who just don't have an awareness of own bodies, there are clinics in Slovenia and Germany that are offering the fasting experience while being monitored by doctors, for complete safety.

The method is very popular today with media people because just a few days of fasting lead to significantly better skin, and the growth hormone improvement also obtained through such therapy leads to a much faster increase in muscle mass after refuelling, thus being popular among performance athletes too. It gives a vigorous impulse to the body, especially a cerebral one. It is recommended to do this method after reading Thierry's book, or after a good doctor's advice, as there are important details to take in consideration, such as: what to firstly eat after fasting; what to expect in day 3, in day 7 and so on; for how long to try it at first depending on your medication, age, etc.

70% of our immune system (our internal doctor) is located in the intestine. Fasting is freeing the doctor from any job other than healing, and what happens is again mind-blowing. Please stay safe with this one and don't force it from the beginning without firstly document yourself! 3 days will give you a nice preview – after 48 hours the DNA gets touched and great things start happening to your body. At the end of fasting, on the first- and second-day, drink only fruit/vegetable juice in order to slowly rebuild the intestinal flora, then continue with light vegan foods for 2-3 days, after which you can return to normal! Even a full day will have some effects. I drank a lot of water during those my fasting, even 7 litres in one day, and did as much physical activity as I could.

Fasting has been used in psychiatric clinics for decades, where no other treatment gave results and the patient was still able to give voluntary consent for it. The outcome is amazing, way more than words can say! It feels like the Windows' function that allows returning to the last healthy state recorded, the back-up function. The mind is sharp and each thought comes in great clarity. It is a huge, overwhelming improvement in thinking and therefore in the behavioural experience!

IV ULTIMATE PHYSICAL EDUCATION

The fitness area is pretty much widely and effectively covered and we all know how important is some sort of sport; I'm sure most of you affected muscularly already have your physiotherapists customising the routine for you. There will be added here **two essential elements: oxygenating the body and cryogenic treatment**.

The simplest way of oxygenating the body is a breathing technique which will surprise by its efficiency. It's **the breathing exercise devised by Wim Hof**, a man who climbed Mount Everest in shorts, a multiple world record holder (for swimming under ice and prolonged full-body contact with ice, for a barefoot half-marathon on ice and snow, etc.), a legend in his field, well-known and easy to be found all-over internet.

The breathing principle is very simple: take 30 big breaths through your nose and after each breath, exhale through your mouth a lower quantity of air than your intake. Then, take a deep breath and exhale; hold until you need to breathe in. Inhale again, as deep as you can, and hold it for 10 seconds. Repeat as many times as you like. This way **oxygen is pushed** to those parts of an inflamed and blocked AS body where oxygen can't get to go easily, including **to the brain**. If you experience a slight dizziness at any point, it means you are performing it correctly. Take it easy at the beginning, maybe even sitting in a chair! Mr. Hof proposes a few more techniques, but only the breathing exercise worked for me and I am recommending. It is a technique scrutinized and approved scientifically as an official gain for the immune system and brain.

This method also helps with being able to make colder and colder showers, when practiced during the shower, and the cold will also have an immediate beneficial impact on the body and also on the mind. Rugby and football players **take an ice bath** after their training

(Cristiano Ronaldo has an ice pool in his living) for fast muscle recovery, so the next day they can train again at full potential. In the same way, a stressed, tense, and strained body under an autoimmune condition, will need this amelioration practice. There are also **gel blankets to be kept in the freezer that can be used again and again on the needed area and the effect is surprising and immediate.** It is good to try only for a few minutes at the beginning, to double-check your sensitivity and the possible compatibility with such a treatment. **In my case, during the period when the decompression of the vertebrae has already started, and physical effort was necessary for the repositioning of the muscles according to the now correct position of the spine, cold therapy was a main friend!**

For those with more money to spare, there are alternative ways to achieve the surplus of oxygen and to get cold treatments: there are **oxygen therapies HBOT, as they are called, where patients enter in a chamber with oxygen at high pressure (hyperbaric)**, the body gets more oxygen, and a mind with enough oxygen functions better, the heart begins to work better and the overall effect against the autoimmune element will improve considerably. The same goes for cryogenic treatments - **cold therapies** where patients are monitored while in a controlled low temperature environment, thus being able to be pushed at their maxim safe limit of supportability, speeding the recovery routine, **with an obvious settling impact on the mind.**

RECOMMENDATIONS

Pushing yourself towards recovery, a little bit every day, at
your own pace, with enthusiasm, is like petrol in a car!
What's in store for us today? It is the mystery of life which
gives us the power! It's the mystery of life which gives the
love to move on!

Everyone has their own mind, with their own recovery time, but right
from the first moment you push your malfunction into healing, the
process becomes a pleasure. It's like setting in motion a train's rusty
wheels: the beginning is the hardest, and then it becomes easier and
easier. Enjoy, keep focused, and don't forget: treat the root of the
problem and not only the effects!

In the US, statistics show that only 30% of people who go to doctors
keep to their prescribed treatment. It's the same here. If you start on the
remission road, do it right, slowly but surely: if you stop you will always
be wondering how it could've been if you'd done things differently. You
could've been healthy by now had you persevered. **It is important to
take responsibility: the necessary vigilance cannot be borrowed!** The
body can be kept in check by the mind when the mind has the whole
rationality, when the rational part masters the irrational part (made of
the five senses and the imagination). When the senses or the imagination
are dominating the mind, the mind is enslaved by passions and loses its
freedom, which is a gift from God, the greatest of all gifts. Someone once
compared the mind with an emperor who has three powers: rationality,
the desire (the explorative spirit, the seeker for good, for personal peace),
and the anger (which is an amplification of the desire, a watch-dog
protecting us from bad when it's turned against our own harmful
passions, and not on other people).

I have tried to keep this book as crisp and svelte as possible, including all vital elements. Besides the bioelectromagnetic clinic, there's not much of an investment. **You can start a new life right now!** It goes without saying that these processes are taking time, maybe the same number of years as the period spent with the disease advancing, but **it's a sure road at your disposal!** Nevertheless, having the full know-how from the beginning will greatly shorten that time for you. The recovery period can be further decreased by a high level of patient involvement.

If I had this book when I was first diagnosed, I reckon I would've had at least 10 more years of health in my life. I wouldn't be who I am today, though. I'm grateful for how things have turned out, for the new wisdom the disease - or, more precisely the recovery from it - revealed. **You have all the directions you need for complete recovery in this book!**

CONCLUSION

After thinking it's all in them and they don't need anyone else, as in Step 1, then shattering their throne, admitting others' existence and wrongly relying on their cheers, as in Step 2, people at Step 3 demand others to love them. At Step 4 they appreciate others to a greater extent but still consider they deserve more, at Step 5 incipient signs of good life appear, people are starting to forgive and flow freely, without strings attached. At Step 6 it's already obvious to them that the more they spread noble joy and good deeds, the more life supports them, and at Step 7 they start to respect and inquire about this good external support as an alive and clever entity guiding them.

After conquering Step 1 people are opening their eyes as if from death, at 2 they reintroduce themselves between others, at 3 they push themselves between others, at 4 is the last step where they still feel they are entitled to a little bit more than the others, at 5 they forgive and become responsible with their game, at 6 they put their souls for others and enjoy the peace life gives them for doing that, and at 7 they understand some higher force is giving them hints, they inquire and discover who's behind it and they become friends with it, understanding that's where peace comes from, together with the authentic forms of love and mental health.

Aiming for reversing the condition and the discipline in following what works are keys. **Mental cleansing** will get rid of inflammatory behaviours, the roots of all bad, and will release the strains in the body created by those roots. The **bioelectromagnetic therapy**, with its correlated diet and natural pills, will free the body from all harmful bacteria and parasites, letting your immune system heal the body, and, most important, freeing the mind from chronic tiredness and helping the mental cleansing. **Fasting** is able to regulate the functions of your glands and organs and will renew you in a mind-blowing manner, especially mentally. **Physical activity, breathing exercises, and cold treatments** are further sharpening the mind so that it can fight at full potential. **Suffering brings patience, patience brings endurance and endurance brings hope. It's not natural for anyone to live without enthusiasm, even while in pain! The pain is there for a reason and, once assuming responsibility, the results of what you will mentally have to do to reverse your autoimmune condition will fill you, on top of physical health, with gratitude and authentic happiness!**

Be good and you'll be good in everything you do!

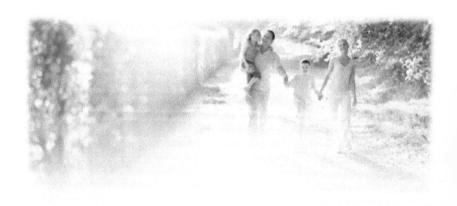

Reference List

- Books:

- *Fasting, by* Thierry de Lestrade
- *Mother Gavrilia, the ascetic of love, by* Nun Gavrilia
- *The Orthodox Way, by* Kallistos Ware
- *The Path to the Kingdom, by* Arsenie Boca

- Donisan, T., Dobrin, M. A., Predeteanu, D., Bojinca, M., Constantinescu, C., Opris, D., Groseanu, L., Borangiu, A., Berghea, F., Balanescu, D., Ionescu, R. and Balanescu, A. (2015), *AB1227-HPR Correlations Between Personality Types, Disease Activity and Quality of Life in Ankylosing Spondylitis (AS) Patients (PTS)*, Annals of the Rheumatic Diseases, pp. 1345.

- Inderjeeth, C., Raymond, W., Connor, C., Edelman, J., Cook, N., Briffa, K. and Mcquade, J. (2016), *AB0670 Ankylosing Spondylitis (AS-P) Patient Centred Education Program Improves Disease Activity and Quality of Life up to 12 Months*, Annals of the Rheumatic Diseases, pp. 1134.

- Keith, L. (2018), *Mental Health Condition linked to Autoimmune Disease*, Autoimmune Disease, Depression, Available at www.managedhealthcareexecutive.com[1], Accessed on 10/10/2019.

- Keith, L. (2018), *Study Evaluates Link Between Stress and Autoimmune Disease*, Autoimmune Disease, Depression,

1. http://www.managedhealthcareexecutive.com

Available at www.managedhealthcareexecutive.com[2], Accessed on 10/10/2019.

- Rogers, M. (1996), *Vibrational Medicine: New Choice for Healing Ourselves (rev. ed.) by Richard Gerber*, Library Journal, Vol.121(10).

- Shmerling, R. H. (2018), *Autoimmune disease and stress, is there a link?* Harvard Health Publishing, Available at www.health.harvard.edu[3], Accessed on 13/11/2019.

- Song, H. (MD, PhD), Fang, F. (MD, PhD), Tomasson, G. (MD, PhD), Amberg, F. (PhD), Mataix-Cols (PhD), D., Fernandez, L. (PhD), Almquist, C. (MD, PhD), Fall, K. (MD, PhD), Valdimarsdottir, U. A. (PhD) (2018), *Association of Stress-Related Disorders with Subsequent Autoimmune Disease*, Jama.

- Upham, B. (2018), *How Stress Affects Ankylosing Spondylitis – and What You Can Do About It?* Available at www.everydayhealth.com[4], Accessed on 7/10/2019.

- Weir, K. (2012), *The roots of mental illness – How much of mental illness can the biology of the brain explain?* Science Watch, Vol. 43, No. 6, Available at www.apa.org[5], Accessed on 20/11/2019.

- Yurdakul, F., Garip, Y., Kocak, R., Almaz, E., Uckun, A. and Bodur, H. (2017), *FRI0439 Psychiatric disorders associated*

---

2. http://www.managedhealthcareexecutive.com

3. http://www.health.harvard.edu

4. http://www.everydayhealth.com

5. http://www.apa.org

with ankylosing spondylitis, Annals of the Rheumatic Disease, Vol. 76, pp. 652.

Appendix 1

FRI0439 Psychiatric disorders associated with Ankylosing Spondylitis

—————— ·|><|]><|· ——————

Background: Ankylosing spondylitis (AS) is an inflammatory rheumatic disease characterized by spinal and/or peripheral involvement, enthesitis, dactylitis, and several extra-articular manifestations. Chronic inflammation often leads to reduced spinal mobility and functional disability. The frequency of fatigue, sleep disturbance, and psychological problems has increased in AS patients (1,2). *Objectives:* Although there are studies investigating depression and anxiety frequency in AS patients, different psychiatric disorders such as impulsivity, alexithymia and eating disorders have not been evaluated. This study aims to investigate the frequency of different psychiatric disorders in AS patients and to evaluate the relationship between these disorders with disease activity and functional status. *Methods:* Patients with AS (n=70) and healthy controls (n=56) were included in the study. The Ankylosing Spondylitis Disease Activity Score (ASDAS), Bath Ankylosing Spondylitis Functional Index, Bath Ankylosing Spondylitis Metrology Index (BASMI), pain visual analog scale, Beck depression scale, Beck anxiety scale, Barrat impulsiveness scale, Toronto alexithymia scale, Eating attitude test, fatigue, Ankylosing spondylitis quality of life, and Nothingam health profile were administered. *Results:* The frequency of depression, anxiety, and non-planning impulsiveness were higher in patients with AS than in healthy controls ($p < 0.05$), although no difference was found in terms of alexithymia, fatigue, and eating attitude. Depression and anxiety were correlated with high disease activity, fatigue, impaired physical functioning, and lower quality of life in the patients with AS. Non-planning impulsiveness was correlated with fatigue and lower quality of life while there was no *correlation with disease activity and functional impairment. BASMI scores were not associated with psychiatric disorders. Table 1. Demographic characteristics and Psychiatric disorders in Ankylosing spondylitis and healthy controls Ankylosing spondylitis patients Healthy controls p——(n=70) (n=56) -—Age (year) 42.85±10.46 44.75±10.04 0.363 Male (%) 57.14% 51.78% 0.548 Beck depression score 13.88±8.99 9.78±8.34 0.006* Beck anxiety score 14.58±10.02 10.53±8.99 0.014* Barrat impulsiveness - attentional score 15.68±3.25 15.21±2.72 0.590 Barrat impulsiveness - motor score 19.62±4.28 18.92±4.23 0.301 Barrat impulsiveness – non-planning score 26.00±4.57 24.78±3.77 0.021* Toronto alexithymia score 54.84±12.86 54.32±11.12 0.644 Eating attitude score 21.74±11.18 22.01±13.24 0.488 *P<0.05.* **Conclusions:** *Depression and anxiety were associated with disease activation, while impulsivity frequency was increased independently of disease activity. Reducing in the quality of life and functional competence due to the psychiatric disorders indicates that, AS patients may require a psychological care approach during the follow-up.'* (Yurdakul et al., 2017)

Appendix 2

AB0670 Ankylosing Spondylitis (AS-P) Patient Centred Education Program Improves Disease Activity and Quality of Life up to 12 Months

— ⟨⟨☒⟩⟩ —

'*Background:* Patient-centred education interventions are rare. After a needs assessment, focus group consultation, and execution of a Plan, Do, Study, Act (PDSA) model, we developed and delivered a multidimensional Ankylosing Spondylitis Education Program (AS-P) to patients referred via a rheumatologist (meeting the New York criteria for AS). **Objectives:** To examine the benefits of AS-P for people with Ankylosing Spondylitis (AS) in regards to health status, quality of life and disease activity. **Methods:** 79 people were recruited in the intervention. Exclusion criteria: 0.05. **Results:** MAFs demonstrated a sustained improvement over 12 months (p=0.011). Similarly, the SF-36 physical (p=0.001) and mental (p=0.002) composite scores had improved 12 months post-intervention. BASFI (p=0.271) and HADs (p=0.086) demonstrated no improvement 12 months post-intervention. **Conclusions:** AS-P for AS is effective in improving AS specific disease activity, pain and QOL scores for up to 12 months.'*
(Inderjeeth et al., 2016)

Appendix 3

AB1227-HPR Correlation Between Personality Types, Disease Activity and Quality of Life in Ankylosing Spondylitis (AS) Patients (PTS)

—— ▭◁▷▭ ——

Background: *AS is a disease with a heavy psychological burden, its main clinical characteristics having a profound impact on health-related quality of life (HRQoL). To study the correlations between personality types, health-related quality of life (HRQoL) and disease activity in SA, few data were available regarding these aspects.* **Methods:** *This cross-sectional study included 90 AS pts from two different Rheumatology Departments (75.6% men, 24.4% women, mean age 43.63, mean duration of disease 12.7 years). Personality types were assessed with Jenkins Activity Survey (JAS-13) for type A/B, State-Trait Anger Expression Inventory Anger-in Scale (AIS) for type C and Type D Personality Scale (DS-14), with its subcomponents (negative affect-NA and social inhibition-SI) for type D. HRQoL was evaluated using the Medical Outcome Study Short-Term-36 (SF36v2), analysing correlations with all subscales (Physical function-PF, Social function-SF, Role physical-RP, Role emotional-RE, Mental health-MH, Vitality-VT, Bodily Pain-BP, Global Health-GH, physical component scores-PCS and mental component scores-MCS). Disease activity was assessed with Bath Ankylosing Spondylitis Disease Activity Index (BASDAI). Analyses were performed using Pearson's correlation coefficients and independent samples t-tests.* **Results:** *Type C pts have lower values of HRQoL components than non-type C (BP t (85) =-2.09, GH t (85) =-2.33, VT t (84)=-2.5, RE t (84)=-2.46, MH t (84)=-2.73, MCS t (84)=-2.61). AIS scores are negatively correlated with all SF36 components (PF r =-0.25, RP r =-0.3, BPr =-0.25, GH r =-0.45, VT r =-0.46, SF r =-0.28, RE r =-0.31, MH r =-0.49, PCS r =-0.26, MCS r*

=-0.42). Furthermore, type C characteristics increased proportionally with BASDAI values (r =0.33). The same negative tendency was noticed for type D pts, with lower overall values for HRQoL (PF t (85)=-1.98, RP t (68.45)=-2.83, BP t (85)=-2.22, GH t (85)=-3.57, VT t (84)=-3.89, SF t (85)=-2.89, RE t (49.77)=-4.2, MH t (84)=5.51, MCS t (84)=-5.2). Furthermore, type D was found to be inversely proportional with HRQoL, where NA was separately correlated with PF r =-0.41, RP r =-0.38, BP r =-0.39, SF r =-0.47 and PCS r =-0.35, and both type D components (NA and SI) correlated with the other HRQoL components (GH rNA =-0.57, rSI =-0.32; VT rNA =-0.61, rSI =-0.35; RE rNA =-0.49, rSI =-0.31; MH rNA =-0.67, rSI =-0.47; MCS rNA =-0.61, rSI =-0.39). Type D individuals have higher BASDAI t (84) =2.42, and type D characteristics increase proportionally with BASDAI (rNA =0.4, rSI =0.22). When compared to type B, type A pts had overall better physical scores and lower disease activity levels. **Conclusions:** Type C and D personalities were found to be strongly correlated with decreased HRQoL and with higher disease activity levels, whereas type A was related to positive results in AS pts. The hypothesis that personality types could influence HRQoL in treatment outcomes should be further analysed. (Donisan et al., 2015)

46

Appendix 4

The diseases appear in the energetic field of people years before they manifest in the physical plan

'The disease comes from the soul and not from the body. Suffering is started upstairs, in the mind, from the conception about the world, from the mental disbalance in which we wander. - Hey, who is narrow in the mind... there's no cure for him! A disease is a red light that tells us we are on a wrong path. If you repeat mistakes for many years, it comes a time of feeling the effects of it - through the disease you created to yourself. In fact, the disease comes because of the loss of the divine element in us, and getting healthy is the result of re-establishing the divine connection. Basically, you heal your body if you firstly heal spiritually. People are made of 3 components: body, soul and spirit, the same with the Wholly Trinity: Father, Son, and Holy Spirit, and a disbalance of any of the 3 components leads to suffering. People who don't believe in God are more exposed to evil, thus to disease. When people infringe the Supreme Laws, weaknesses in the defence mechanisms appear, the immune system fails, so they become an easy prey for viruses, becoming sick. People who believe are mentally and physically stronger than those who don't. The road to healing is the road to God. All the diseases are self-created and the doctors finally catch up with understanding it. The diseases appear in the energetic field of people years before they manifest in the physical plan.'
(Boca, 1989)

Appendix 5

Bioelectromagnetic Therapy
Doctor RIFE and the resonant frequency

———$\blacktriangleright\mathbb{C}\mathbb{D}\mathbb{C}$———

'Around 1930, in Sant Diego, scholar-doctor Raymond Royal Rife started looking for solutions against cancer. His first invention was the Universal Rife Microscope, which could enlarge living cells, bacteria and viruses up to 30,000 times. Rife then soon discovered each organism has own resonant frequency. With a bacteria sample under the microscope, Rife used to operate a frequency generator which was producing an electromagnetic field in conjunction with bacteria's frequency. After a few minutes, all the bacteria stopped moving and died. Rife then started using the discovery on people and could destroy ordinary bacteria, cure chronic infections and fight even with hard diseases using the principle the vibrational resonance. Rife could destroy viruses and bacteria as easy as you can break a glass using the resonance principle (such the big opera singer Caruso did). Rife observed severe diseases are caused by a group of viruses and micro-organisms generically called BX. He discovered the resonant frequency needed to address them and made laboratory tests on animals. All viruses and micro-organisms had disintegrated and animal cured. From here the technology started being used on people too. Doctor Rife was not the only researcher experimenting with the use of an electromagnetic field in curing diseases. George Lakhovky was also using his Multiple Waves Oscillator in curing most serious illnesses.' (Rogers, 1996)

About the author

J King

♣

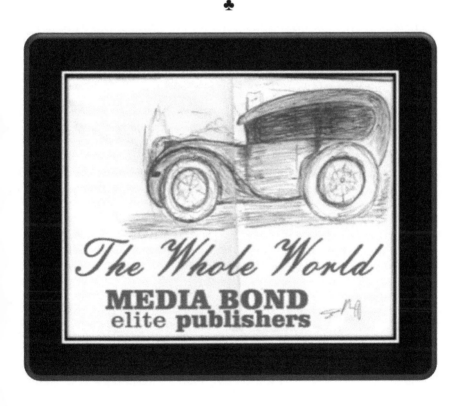

♣

After 13 years of Ankylosing Spondylitis (AS) 'prison', J King won the fight against the disease with no cure in the medicine of 2019 and concentrated in his books the Eureka results of the tens of thousands of hours invested in discovering and changing the harmful behaviours that led him to almost dying.

A former martial arts national champion, he used self-control to understand the body, tested himself in a wide variety of biological and psychological experiments, monitored and gathered results as a full-time activity. During the first years with AS he tried to unnaturally keep a body posture, wrongly thinking that this is going to make him healthy. It didn't help, it brought even more pain and mental stress, but it offered unprecedented awareness and understanding of the anatomy. He can now individually unstrain his muscles, even the peripheral ones, he can feel all tensions in the body and went as far as being able to link them with the moods and behaviours that are producing them, leading to the amazing discoveries he brought to public's attention with his books.

People from all over the world are now becoming healthy not only physically, but also mentally, as a result of reading and using the instruments and solutions presented in J King's collection. His unrivalled research is a gift not only to those suffering from autoimmune diseases but to the entire world, his findings being able to reveal fixes in all aspects and areas of life, leading, as bold as it sounds, to ultimate happiness!

MEDIA BOND elite publishers

Praise for the author

People really are amazing. I am so grateful I came across J King's books. They are as my best friends now!

- Emily. Facebook

9 798201 089764